WHAT WOULD
FLO DO?

A REAL-WORLD GUIDE FOR THE
NEW NURSE PRECEPTOR

Rachel Edmondson, BHA, BSN, RN-BC

Cover created by Katie Swaim Design

Ordering Information
Quantity sales: Special discounts are available on quantity purchases by corporations, associations, and others. For details, contact the publisher at the above email address.

Printed in the United States of America.
ISBN 13: 978-0-9981114-3-8
ISBN 10: 0-9981114-3-0

Disclaimer
The information provided herein is stated to be truthful and consistent, in that any liability, in terms of inattention or otherwise, by any usage or abuse of any policies, processes, or directions contained within is the solitary and utter responsibility of the recipient reader. Under no circumstances will any legal responsibility or blame be held against the publisher for any reparation, damages, or monetary loss due to the information herein, either directly or indirectly.

The information herein is offered for informational purposes solely, and is universal as so. The presentation of the information is without contract or any type of guarantee assurance.

The trademarks that are used are without any consent, and the publication of the trademark is without permission or backing by the trademark owner. All trademarks and brands within this book are for clarifying purposes only and are owned by the owners themselves, not affiliated with this document.

CONTENTS

This book is dedicated to the OG preceptors of mine who taught me everything I know, Alli Ramsey and Cara Johnston. Your patience, your kindness, and the knowledge you imparted on me in my early career are unforgettable. You taught me that it's OK to laugh. Juice breaks are crucial to surviving a 12-hour shift. And feeding an NPO patient before surgery is probably not the best idea. Thank you for showing me the beauty of our profession. I am forever grateful.

Introduction to Nurse Tribe

Everyone needs a tribe, an instinctual community and family with like purpose. Bound together by common dialect, intention, and social likeness, welcome to Nurse Tribe. Our dialect is human touch and the power of medicine. Our purpose is the protection and healing of humankind. Our likeness is compassion, grace, and service.

Carefully curated by nurses to educate and inspire, Nurse Tribe offers a place of solitude, of connectedness, of raw, unfiltered—sometimes grammatically incorrect—candidness about navigating a world that misunderstands the magic of what we do. As an affiliate of Nurseology, an Austin-based company that sells products for nurses, our mission is to further strengthen our tribe's fabric by building community through continuing education, experience, and relevant discussion.

Follow us on Instagram @thenursetribe or at www.thenursetribe.org as we chronicle our own experiences in nursing and strive to empower our community!

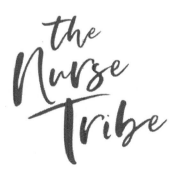

LOOK AT YOU, STUD

Rumor has it that you have been asked to be a nurse preceptor. Kinda crazy, right? Maybe, you are thinking *why me? Am I really cut out for this?* Let's just stop that negative self-talk right here and put those feelings to bed because here's the thing: Your manager or educator saw something in you that made her believe you are up for a new challenge. And this challenge is huge, friend. Precepting is a giant undertaking that ain't for the faint of heart. Why? You ask. Let's explore this a little deeper.

I want you to think back to when you were a new nurse. There were *a lot* of feelings. Remember that overwhelming feeling of failing, making a mistake, losing your license, and ending up selling tiki drinks at a retirement village in Florida? Or was that just me? Maybe your fears were not that extreme, but I can almost guarantee that all new nurses experience a version of the same fears.

What will happen if _____?

You can fill in the blank with just about anything, and it is probable that a new nurse sitting somewhere in this world has likely experienced that very same fear in some form or fashion.

Here's the good news. You—yes, you, nurse preceptor—can ultimately change the shape of history for these new graduate nurses. How? By validating those fears and carefully molding the nurse you precept into the nurse you want to work along side of. And this book is here to help you do just that.

From how to handle the *overly-anxious-by-the-book-this-isn't-how-we-learned-it-in-nursing-school* new graduate to constructively giving feedback to a new nurse who just isn't quite grasping core concepts, this book is a whirlwind of pro tips and tricks to help you lead a new nurse through the most impressionable first few weeks of her new job.

Drawing from real-world nursing scenarios and *wish-I-woulda'-done-that* lightbulb moments from my own precepting practice, this book aims to help you best utilize the short time frame you have to get a new nurse practicing independently at the bedside. And given the costly nature of training nurses, it's my bet your organization expects you to work your magic at lightening speed.

So let's get down to business. I've skipped some of the evidence (sorry to all the academics smiting me right now), and made this a down-and-dirty practical guide to being a *boss* preceptor in the messy real world of nursing. It's time for you to use this book to take on the next challenge of your nursing career. I know it can be scary. I know it can be tough. But here we are, and it's time to use your knowledge, strengths, and experiences to shape the next generation of nurses at the bedside. And trust you may learn something about yourself along the way.

THE NITTY-GRITTY

As a preceptor, you have been charged with providing a valuable learning experience that immerses a new graduate into bedside nursing as seamlessly as possible. It's a huge responsibility that requires you to know the basics of your organization's orientation process. It is your job to know and understand what is expected of you as a preceptor, and this should be clearly defined by the facilitator of the orientation, be it your educator or manager. From paperwork requirements to achievement milestones, as a preceptor, you need to be clear on several items before your embark on this adventure with your new graduate nurse. Let's get this boring stuff out of the way so we can move on to the fun stuff in the following chapters.

The Need-to-Know Boring-Stuff

- The length of orientation is important to nail down. Why? It gives you a time frame that helps create a necessary framework for orientation.

  - Finding out how long the orientation period is allows you to plan accordingly. Later on in this book, you will learn how to strategically (and safely) increase your orientee's patient assignment so that by the end of orientation, he is practicing independently at the bedside.

- Determine when the orientee's first day on the unit will be and if she will be following your schedule. Most organization's orientation process involves a combination of both classes and shift work with one or two preceptors.

  - Let's be honest: surprises are never good in nursing. Find out when exactly the new nurse starts on the unit.

Whoever is managing orientation schedules should have the exact start dates so that you can get organized and be prepared.

- Find out the paperwork requirements for being a preceptor. I would bet my next paycheck that it will be a boatload. By having a clear understanding of what paperwork you will be required to complete for your orientee, you will waste no time backtracking or trying to remember when he accomplished certain skills.

  - Although each organization is different, it is likely you will have an electronic or paper core competency packet that must be completed by the end of the orientation period. These competencies vary per unit but often involve care milestones such as verifying the nurse is competent in tracheostomy care or interpreting 12-lead EKGs. Knowing these competencies can help you set weekly goals for your orientee and can provide a framework for orientation.

  - You may also be responsible for weekly or biweekly status reports on your orientee's performance. Relax! I would never leave you hanging. There is a whole chapter on feedback later in the book.

- Verify what your organization's policy is on charting. How do you verify your orientee's charting during shift? Is it assumed that you reviewed it? Do you put in a nurse's note? Is there a verify function in your electronic record? Get these questions answered ahead of time!

So Ima' stop right here and move on to the juicy stuff. If you are a nurse who is going to be precepting, you have more than likely completed an orientation of your own that will be in some ways similar to the orientation of the RN you are precepting. Being prepared and understanding expectations is the driving point here. Mmmmkay?

THE FIRST DATE

Even though orientation periods differ per unit, organization, and specialty, it is likely that your organization has paired you with an orientee whom you will spend a lot of one-on-one time with over the next several months. Hopefully, you will be matched with someone with which your manager or educator feels is a good fit for you personality-wise (you mesh well together). This relationship will grow respectively over time, but the first shift can be especially awkward. Be prepared! You are entering the equivalent of a blind-date situation of which you have work-through on your own. Check out my advice on how to navigate the **DOs** and **DONTs** for your very first shift with your orientee.

DO

- Find out your orientee's phone number and shoot her a text message the night before her first shift. This is especially important if you have not had a chance to meet her in person.
- Ensure that your orientee has a copy of your patient assignment when she arrives in the morning (care cards, Kardex).
- Introduce her to *everyone*. Remember how it feels to be the new gal on the block? Use your manners, friend.
- Over the course of the first day, make sure she has access to:
  - Pyxis or ADC
  - Computer system
  - Electronic medical record

- Together, walk through your supply room, break room, nutrition room, and workstations.
- Have your orientee write down important numbers including:
  - Charge nurse
  - Unit secretary
- Explain to her the process of having to call in sick or who to call if she is running late. Yes, we are all human.
- Ask your orientee how she learns best. This will be helpful in tailoring your teaching style ahead of time.
- Manage expectations *right now*. Explain that you need to verify competence in even the most baby of nursing tasks before allowing her to fly solo in all aspects of nursing care. More on this later in the book.
- If you skipped the first step (tsk tsk), exchange numbers with your orientee at the end of your first shift. This will no doubt come in handy.

DON'T

- Give him patients on his very first day. Allow him to observe the flow of the unit and navigate where things are before making him jump right in. Remember this is a marathon, not a sprint.
- Trust him without verifying he is competent in a skill or task. This is a rule of thumb throughout the entirety of nursing orientation, and it begins on the first day.
- Be afraid to delegate on the first day. After you have seen him safely take a patient to the restroom or hang a medication, it is OK to start pushing independence early.
- Expect to leave work right at the end of your shift. From here on out, friend, your night or day just got a hair longer and you need to be OK with this. It is your responsibility to make

sure that care is safely passed to the oncoming nurse, documentation is complete, and action items are finished regardless of who is primarily caring for the patient.

WWFD (What Would Flo Do)?

My girl Flo once said, "The most important practical lesson that can be given to nurses is to teach them what to observe." Do just that. Observation is integral to the nursing process. You can learn almost anything simply through observation. Begin to engrain this way of thinking on the very first day!

BABY STEPS

It should not go without mentioning that the first four weeks of orientation are the most difficult part of precepting. Why? Because you will spend these shifts working almost double what you are used to, and this is for several reasons.

The new nurse is GREEN, GREEN, GREEN.

It is important to remember that your orientee's last contact with a patient was probably in the ballpark of two to three months before her first shift on the unit. To boot, you don't know what her nursing school experience was like! Some schools have capstone semesters, whereas others have clinical only one day a week up until the last semester. Because the complexity of patient care in nursing school varies, you must remember that you are essentially building the orientee as a nurse from the ground up with very little real-world experience.

What does this mean? It is your responsibility to verify that the nurse graduate can perform the most basic of nursing tasks. The key here is to never assume that an orientee knows how to do something; always ask about his comfort level and then verify his competence in the task at hand. From setting up suction to administering insulin, it is your responsibility to watch him do a skill before you allow him to perform the task (no matter how small) on his own. I suggest that you make this clear from the very first shift. Help the orientee understand that it is not to micromanage, but rather to be sure he can do a skill correctly and safely, and that he doesn't have any questions.

The orientee has to learn WORKFLOW.

In addition to verifying competency in performing certain tasks, your orientee will have to learn how the unit ebbs and flows. Use the very first shift as a "shadow day." This allows you to work out any kinks (ensuring she has computer access, knows the floor layout) and gives you a chance to point out how your unit runs on any given day.

How does your unit ebb and flow? Answer these questions for the orientee:
- When do the most transfers happen?
- When do most discharges happen?
- When do nurses take breaks?
- When do most physicians round?
- When do the majority of admissions happen?
- When are most medications due?
- Which part of charting takes the most time?
- What are the charting requirements for the floor?

Answering these questions will help your orientee tailor her patient care in an efficient manner, and it creates a rough timeline that helps her fine-tune her nursing practice.

The orientee has to learn the WHY behind the WHAT.

In addition to explaining how to do various tasks, the first several weeks of orientation seem rather drawn out because you are having to be a nurse *and* explain in great detail the gravity of the *why* behind *what* you are doing. You do this in

15

an effort to help the new nurse develop thought behind his actions so that he is not just mindlessly checking off tasks. By explaining why you are doing something, you are prompting your orientee to critically think about his actions at all times.

Tasks that could take you normally 5 minutes to complete will now take you 20. Report that normally takes you 30 minutes may now take you 45. But it's not for any other reason than to strategically prepare your orientee for the day she is off orientation and you are no longer there to remind her why someone admitted for syncopal episodes should ever be left alone in the bathroom. Get ma' drift?

WWFD?

As you precept, remember that you are essentially shaping an RN that you will eventually work *with* at the bedside. Do you want an RN working alongside of you that knows only shortcuts? Or someone you can rely on to watch your patients when you step away from the bedside for lunch? This is up to you, and if Flo were here today, I think she would agree.

Support her. Mold her. Help her be the best nurses she can be.

THE STRUGGLE IS REAL: TIME MANAGEMENT

Just as you and I once did, it is safe to say that almost all new graduate nurses struggle with time management. You must remember that they are going from 0 to 90 in roughly 10 to 16 weeks. Remember nursing school? The days when you got to care for patients without shouldering the entire burden of care? Those days are gone! And it is up to you to help school your orientee in the world of time management. This requires *a lot* of feedback, coaching, and prompting, which I'll cover in a hot minute.

Time management is a beast and probably the most frustrating part of any nurse's new gig. Why? She's more than likely been a high performer her whole life and wholeheartedly, with every ounce of her being, believes she is a fast learner (and she probably is). The difference is that this time she is learning in an unpredictable, semichaotic environment that throws 100 apples her way and expects her to make lemonade. Amirite?

So how do you go about helping the orientee tackle this so-called beast? It's a complex process that involves a 12-hour itinerary, short-term goal setting, and constant shuffling of priorities based on the apples aiming in the direction of one's forehead.

The 12-hour Itinerary

The first step in helping an orientee master time management is to provide him with a generic hour-by-hour timeline of a typical day on your unit. I'm talking a *"roses are red, violets are blue kinda"* day where everything seems to fall into place.

Here is an example of my day.

0630–0645: Get assignment. Look up patient labs/read 1 physician note
0645–0655: Shift update/huddle (whatever you call it)
0655–0730: Hand-off
0730–0745: Fill in gaps needed to complete patient picture
0745–1130: 5 patient assessments & notes charted & all AM meds passed
1030–1200: Patient rounding (check-ins) & discharge surge
1200–1300: Miscellaneous tasks & afternoon med pass
1300–1330: Lunch
1330–1400: Charting
1400–1600: Patient rounding, more discharges, miscellaneous tasks, outstanding charting
1600–1800: Expected transfers, evening meds, final charting
1800: Final patient rounds before shift change
1850: Hand-off

By providing an itinerary from takeoff to crash landing (hopefully not), you are helping "chunk" patient care into a series of short-term goals. Let's break this down a little bit more.

This perfect day in nursing paradise should include a schedule with time frames of when you prefer to have things accomplished by. To this very day, no matter the patient load, I aim to have my assessments charted and all morning medications passed by 1000, lunch by 1330, and miscellaneous charting completed by 1500. These time frames were taught to me by my preceptor almost five years ago, and I can count on *one* of my hands how many times I have stayed late to complete unfinished charting. By helping your orientee form this habit early on, you are keeping her caught up at all times should an emergency rise.

Reprioritization

Mmmmk, Rachel, but what if it *isn't* a perfect day and these "goals" you speak of are not practical? Great question! It's important to communicate to your orientee that patient safety, emergencies, timely medications, and other such important tasks and events take priority over charting and the day-to-day minutia of one's shift.

Always.No.Matter.What.

Helping your orientee incorporate this practice into reality will involve reprioritization of her nursing care and a simple retiming of her goals. For instance, let's say that during one of your shifts together, you have been in a room of a crumping patient for two hours of your morning and it's now 0930. Your orientee still has medications to pass in all three of her other rooms and an admission on the way. Having assessments charted and meds passed by 1000 is just probably not going to happen at this point, correct?

Here's what you do:
- The two of you need to first take five minutes for yourselves. Go to the break room or nutrition room, and have a juice break. You read that correctly. Juice can make anything better, and it comes highly recommended by Yours Truly. But for real—it gives you a minute to decompress, breathe, and raise your blood sugar.
- After said juice break, have your orientee list pending action items in order of most important to least important.

19

Don't do this for him. Caught ya' mama-birding a little, didn't I? It is so important that he walks you through this. Ask him *calmly* what he would do first, next, and so on.

- *Softly* correct him if you need to, but help him think it through. Ask him why he would choose to do Y over X to help understand his way of thinking.
- Now take your to-do list and help your orientee set a new itinerary. What is the new time frame for having assessments charted and medications passed? When are you going to aim to grab lunch?

It's important to mention that even if an emergency doesn't cause a hiccup in your plan, something else can. The idea of always expecting the worst needs to be communicated with your orientee. Perhaps you have a new admission right at shift change, two discharges to complete, or a very talkative patient who is demanding quite a bit of attention. There are many hiccups that can be encountered during the day—as you are, I'm sure, aware—and it is crucial to highlight the constant restructuring of one's day based once again on the apples thrown in your direction.

Regardless, having a similar routine during each shift is the key to success in nursing. I try to instill this practice in every new nurse I precept, as I believe it is a sure fire way to stay on task and maintain efficiency throughout the entire shift.

WWFD?

Well, she wrote this poem for you.
You are a nurse
So, expect the worst
But if you always chart first
You'll never be cursed.

MAMA BIRD

Gone are the days of "nurses eating their young." You are about to enter a sacred relationship that will have you slashing the tires of the first person who yells at your orientee. OK, perhaps not that extreme. But I promise there is something very personal about the preceptor–orientee relationship. Your orientee depends on you to support her. Protect her. And allow her to spread her wings when it's time to fly.

So let's talk about you and yours for a moment and taking flight. If you are new to the precepting game, which presumably you are because you purchased this book, there is a delicate balance when it comes to the baby bird leaving the nest, the orientee flying solo. I've seen and have had to coach preceptors that have been all over the spectrum when it comes to mama-birding. From micromanaging to allowing an orientee to sink before teaching her to swim, let's review a rough timeline to help you gauge how involved you should be throughout the trajectory of nursing orientation.

The Mama-Bird Timeline

Week 1: The Wicked Tight Grip

Verify everything, including your orientee's basic skills; do almost all menial tasks for the orientee; catch new graduate up when he is behind; take report and assist in giving report; call physicians; talk the most in patient rooms; prioritize for the orientee; give feedback.

Weeks 2 and 3: The Brunt of Orientation Work

Assist the new nurse with things she has never done before; remind orientee of pending action items; let orientee take the reins in patient rooms; allow new nurse to pass medications on her own (but you may quiz her first); listen to nurse give and take report; guide orientee on how to pick up her pace; insist orientee page physicians (but be close by to interject if needed); help nurse plan talking points before calling MD; jump in when orientee is in over her head; give RN feedback.

Weeks 4-6: The Loose Grip

Assist orientee with things he has never done before; wait slightly longer to remind new nurse of pending action items (testing knowledge); allow orientee to fly *almost* solo in patient rooms; expect RN to page physicians without being present; still discuss why orientee is paging physicians; help new nurse navigate challenging situations; give feedback.

Weeks 6-8: First Flight

Assist orientee with things she has never done before; let some of the pending, noncritical to-dos be late so that orientee understands the cascade affect of poor time management; expect nurse to fly solo in patient rooms; expect orientee to page physicians without prompting; help orientee critically think through questions by not giving the answers; give feedback.

Weeks 8-10: Leaving the Nest

Assist orientee with things he has never done before; remind nurse of priorities; expect orientee to take a full patient assignment and be the boss of patient care; give feedback.

Nursing orientation is a delicate balance of freedom and collaboration between you and your orientee that involves trust, safety, and honest communication. That being said, let's look a little closer at how to manage an orientee's patient ratio throughout nursing orientation.

PATIENT RATIO

When I served in an interim educator role, new preceptors always had one burning question, "Rachel, How do I safely increase my orientee's patient load throughout orientation?" This might be the very reason you purchased this book, and I want to make an important disclaimer before we jump into the heart of the matter.

Not.Every.Orientee.Is.The.Same.

There, I said it. We all learn in different ways, and each of us has a unique response to the structure of nursing orientation. There are some new nurses that just *get it* and fly solo pretty early on. Others are just over there on Week 10 of orientation afraid to put one foot in front of the other. It is important to recognize this and to adjust accordingly. There is no reason to keep someone at two patients on Week 3 of orientation when she is truly ready to advance to taking three.

For the purposes of this chapter, we are going to assume the nurse:patient ratio is 5:1 on a high-acuity medical floor and orientation is 10 weeks long. If you are working within a different specialty or have a different length of orientation, try to adjust the numbers accordingly.

The Generic *Rx*

	Patient Load	Acuity
Week 1	Take 1 patient	1st shift = shadow day 2nd shift = 1 easy patient

	Patient Load	Acuity
Week 2	Take 1-2 patient(s)	Easiest/simple patient(s): No admissions/open rooms* No possible transfer orders* No possible discharge orders*
Week 3	Take 1-2 patient(s)	Easiest/simple patient(s) No admissions/open rooms* No possible transfer orders* No possible discharge orders*
Week 4	Take 2-3 patients	2-3 easiest patients (leave higher acuity for next week) 2 patients staying on unit and 1 open bed
Week 5	Take 3 patients	2 easier patients and 1 higher acuity/complex patient 3rd patient can be an admission/discharge/transfer*
Week 6	Take 3-4 patients	3 easier patients and 1 higher acuity/complex patient Transition to 4th patient at end of the week*

	Patient Load	Acuity
Week 7	Take 4 patients	2 easier patients and 2 higher acuity/complex patients
Week 8	Take 4-5 patients	Transition to full patient load at beginning of the week
Week 9	Take 5 patients	Take full load
Week 10	Take 5 patients independently	Take full load

Adapted from PCU Graduate Nurse Guide to Unit Orientation, Stephanie Franks, 2017

Side note: Take report on all of your patients and decide after report which patients are higher versus lower acuity, and which ones will probably leave the unit via transfer or discharge by the end of the day, and sort out your open bed situation.

Additionally, high acuity can mean a number of things:
- More complex r/t tube feedings, total care, and other tasks
- Demanding patient or family
- Closer patient monitoring, and other patient needs

Phew, that's a lot of information! Remember that this is not a one size fits all, but simply a guide to help you efficiently advance your orientee's patient ratio each week. Now, let's answer all those "buts" I can hear you screaming at me through the page.

But ... my orientee feels like she isn't ready.

News flash, friend: no one ever feels ready. If I could have stayed on orientation for six months, I woulda'! There is a lot of anxiety that comes with nursing orientation, and it is important that you help your orientee understand that there is a difference between her perception of her performance and her actual performance.

Your job as a preceptor is to safely push your orientee's boundaries while simultaneously offering support and encouragement. How would you encourage your orientee to try to place a Foley if he is uncomfortable with that skill? By explaining the process, assisting him through it, and praising him when he successfully completes the task. In just the same manner, it's time to push him to take that additional patient.

Now, let me be clear: a true safety concern or performance issue will blatantly be staring you in the face and needs to be addressed immediately with whoever is facilitating your unit's orientation.

But … my orientee had a bad shift.

I cannot tell you how many times I have had preceptors tell me that they are "bumping" their orientee back down to a smaller patient load because she had a bad shift. Nine times out of ten this so-called bad day was the first time the orientee increased her patient load, let's say from two patients to three patients. What you must remember is that she is now having to rework her patient care timelines and workflow with an additional patient to care for. Therefore, orientees are likely to have a harder day each time they increase their patient load. Explain this to your orientee ahead of time in an effort to manage her expectations.

Shift.Happens.Amirite?

For that extra-bad shift where nothing seemed to go right, it is your job as a preceptor to be positive and supportive. Reflect on what went right together at the end of shift and where things went wrong. This is crucial to your orientee's development and confidence as a nurse. By decreasing his patient load, you are solidifying a message that he, in fact, is not capable, and his confidence will suffer.

There are times for learning, and there are times for stepping in. We want all of our new grads to have experience paging doctors, speaking with family members, and just plain figuring it out. But if your patient begins crumping, consider stepping in. You really don't need your orientee fumbling through an SBAR with an MD on the phone if a patient needs to be transferred to ICU. She needs clear, experienced help sometimes—that is when it is time to step in. The same applies with an upset or irate family member. Remember, the orientee probably has never experienced this before and might not know how to necessarily maneuver through the situation.

WWFD

Florence once brilliantly stated, "So never lose an opportunity of urging a practical beginning, however small, for it is wonderful how often in such matters the mustard-seed germinates and roots itself."

Start small. Start practical. Watch them grow.

SAYING NO: CUTTING THE SMALL-TASK CORD

All right, Mama Bird. When you are precepting, it is easy to get caught up doing small tasks for your orientee. They are the behind-the-scenes nursing and non-nursing action items that must get done for our patients. But they also require prioritization for adequate time management.

What are these tasks?
- Collecting labs
- Taking patients to the restroom
- Dressing changes
- Starting a new IV
- Replacing an empty fluid bag
- Giving pain medicine
- Finding an SCD machine
- Completing an admission screen
- Rechecking a blood pressure
- Tracking down a medication
- Getting an EKG

The list is endless, but these are the tasks that require learning how to appropriately cluster care and effectively use your resources. During the first few weeks of orientation, you will probably be performing a lot of these types of tasks in the background for your orientee. But as the weeks progress, it is vital that you assist your orientee in learning how and where to acquire supplies, whom to call when a certain issue needs troubleshooting, and how to effectively cluster care when a bunch of small tasks need to be completed.

About halfway through orientation, it is important that you ultimately stop completing these tasks for your orientee. It may seem harsh, but it is vital that your orientee understands how time consuming these menial tasks can be, and that she learns how to navigate and troubleshoot on her own. So, Mama Bird, it's time to softly say no. How? Let's look at the following scenario.

It's 11 p.m., and your new grad is currently in a patient room completing an assessment. One of his other patients is calling for pain medication. And he has an IV beeping because he let a bag of fluids run dry in 404. He calls you asking if you could medicate his patient for pain or go see why the IV is beeping in 404. Also 403 needs to use the bathroom. "Please help!" he says.

Stop! Before you drop what you are doing and complete the tasks for him, have him come meet you in the hallway. Let's walk him through this.

You: Let's look at the tasks you need to complete.
Orientee: Toilet a patient, give a pain pill, troubleshoot an IV.
You: What are you doing right now?
Orientee: Finishing up an assessment.
You: Is this something you can come back to in a moment?
Orientee: Yes, but I want to get it done, and I figured since you were here …
You: Mark, I'm not always going to be here. What would you do if I wasn't here? Who would you call? What could you delegate?
Orientee: I could call the tech to help the patient to the restroom.

You: OK, perfect. Then what?

Orientee: I could run in and replace the bag of fluids really quick and then go medicate my other patient for pain. Then I'll finish my assessment.

You: Perfect. Get started!

That was a great soft no, Mama Bird! I know it was hard, but it is important to get your orientee in the mindset that you are not always going to be around to save the day! He has to learn how to effectively delegate and manage the "small stuff" on his own. I know it feels like you are abandoning him, but you are really only preparing him for the day he gets off of orientation.

The last few weeks, especially, are essential in cutting that small-task cord! You can soften the blow by managing your orientee's expectations at the beginning of your shift. Explain that you are not trying to be mean, but that your hands-off behavior is crucial to his success after orientation.

WWFD: How to Say No, Like Flo the Pro

- Who would you call if I wasn't here?
- Can you delegate anything right now?
- I'm not going to be here in a few weeks, and I want you to understand how to manage small tasks and prioritize.
- I am here to support you today, but you are doing so well on your own that I am only jumping in if you really need me.

Preceptor Responsibilities

Look at you, Papa Bear. It's Week 5 of orientation, and your orientee is independently taking three patients and managing her patients' care with little prompting. Way to kill that preceptor game!

Now, I have some questions for you:
What medications did your orientee pass this morning on Mr. Smith in 205?
What was the recent potassium for the patient in 208?
What is the discharge plan for 202?

Can you answer these questions? You better be able to, nurse friend. As a preceptor, you are responsible for all of the patients you are assigned *even* once your orientee is taking the full patient load. Yes, she is a licensed body. Yes, your new nurse is "prettyish" independent, but you are essentially supervising her and the care that she is providing to each patient. You must be in the know on all of your patients. You never know when an emergency will happen or when you will be called upon to answer questions that are crucial to your patient outcomes.

Tips for Staying Up-to-Date Without Hovering

- Listen to and receive report on all of your patients alongside your orientee regardless of how far into orientation she is.
- Introduce yourself to each patient *after* your orientee has met and introduced herself. If you are completing bedside shift report, ensure she dominates the conversation and introductions. This will occur over time as comfort increases, but it is crucial to let her have the first words. It

is the only way to establish trust between a patient and a nurse in training.

- While your orientee is completing her assessments, take this time to look up the most recent prog notes, medications, and labs, and review all orders.
- Complete any pertinent assessment observations for any patient that is higher acuity or unstable. Ensure your assessment data match your orientee's.
- If you see an MD in the hall, *find your orientee*. It is very easy to touch base with the doctor while you have him there. But hold your tongue, Chatty Kathy! If at all possible, politely say, "Let me get the nurse taking care of the patient. She can probably tell you a little bit more."

THE FEEDBACK LOOP

Feedback plays an essential role in the success of an orientee. Some of you are squirming in your seat just reading that sentence, but I am here to offer you some help when it comes to giving your orientee a *swift kick in the reality department* should he need it.

The truth is this: you must give feedback.

And this is probably the hardest part of being a preceptor. Crucial conversations are just that—crucial! The thing that you must remember is that your orientee is likely craving feedback, positive or negative. We all want to know where we stand when starting a new job; new nurses are no different! Feedback on progress, both good and bad, is vital to their success.

Pearls of Wisdom: Real-Time Feedback

- Construct your feedback sandwich. Layer feedback by utilizing the "good, constructive, good" method.
- Seek permission to give feedback. Start the conversation by asking if you can share something that might help your orientee be safer, save time, and generally thrive. This helps him understand that you have observed an action, and you want to offer an alternative way of doing the same thing.
- Share your concern in private. Not in a patient room, a busy hallway, or other public space. Use your nursing judgement here.
- Share your concern in a compassionate way. Your orientee is likely going to be mortified that he made a

mistake or compromised safety. Remember to keep your feedback centered on the actual problem; these conversations are best served succinctly.

Pearls of Wisdom: After-Shift Feedback

- This must be done every shift. Period. It doesn't always have to be a long and drawn-out conversation. I like having short feedback discussions as we are walking to our cars.
- This short conversation should start by having your orientee recognize a win (something she did really well) and then follow up that recognition and praise with one question that is your feedback knockout:

"What do you feel you could have done differently today?"

This question is a game changer! Why? It forces your orientee to introspectively think about her performance. Using this tactic allows her to tell you where her performance deficit lies. Every time I use this feedback mechanism, the orientee names whatever it is he or she needs my coaching on, whether it's time management, confidence when speaking to team members or patients, or any number of actions.

- Ask your orientee to name one thing she learned that she did not know before. It is a great practice that will keep orientees humble.
- Limit the praise if you feel as though your orientee will *not* hear the constructive aspect of the conversation.
- Before you leave for the day, set some realistic goals together for your next shift. This is a great way to utilize the *"What do you feel you could have done differently?"* conversation. Perhaps your orientee needs to work on

speeding up the time spent in patient's rooms, communicating with family or doctors, or increasing the speed of charting. Use her struggle to set a goal for the next shift.

SUSIE, SAM, AND CATHY

After the first week jitters wear off, it is likely you will be able to determine the personality type of your orientee pretty quickly.

Having precepted gaggles of baby nurses, I have used my own experiences to compile a little advice to help you navigate some of the more difficult personalities you may encounter. Remember, this is not a one-size-fits-all approach, but it may help you effectively navigate some more challenging situations.

Overly Anxious Susie

Susie. She thinks everything is an emergency. An infiltrated IV might cause her to think her patient is going to lose his arm. She lacks confidence, but her knowledge is there. Her assessments take her 30 minutes per patient. She asks questions that she knows the answers to. One hiccup in the shift will cause her to derail for hours. She will do anything and everything for all of her patients, which makes time management a very difficult feat. Oh, and if you didn't guess it already, she struggles with delegation.

How to Deal
- Remain calm. Always. Soft, direct communication is key with Susie. She can get worked up very easily, so an understanding, kind approach is best.
- Reinforce her strengths. Susie is typically a very smart new nurse who remembers everything she studied in nursing school. She is very detail oriented, and her assessments are

exceptionally thorough. Use this as the "good" part of your feedback sandwich.

- Try to avoid giving feedback to Susie in front of her patients. Correct any safety issues immediately, but any in-depth discussion should be reserved for one-on-one feedback outside (this is appropriate across the board).

- When she is behind, it is important to help her understand her list of pending priorities. Be straightforward. Tell her she is behind and needs to move on to the next thing. She needs direction and reminders in this area. Likely, she is caught up in a room doing a task that can be delegated or is not a priority in that particular moment. Remember, softness is key during this conversation.

- Ask her how she is feeling often and validate her feelings of anxiety. Help her understand that what she is experiencing is normal but needs to be worked through. If she is starting to get worked up in front of a patient, bring her outside the room and take a minute to decompress. A juice break comes in handy here!

Slowpoke Sam

Sam. Oh, Sam. He mainly struggles with assessments and his morning medication passes. It's usually noon by the time he finishes his assessments and morning medications. His sense of urgency is practically nonexistent. He has trouble clustering care. Watching him walk back and forth out of the supply room has become part of your morning ritual.

How to Deal

- First, you must understand that Sam is more than likely worried about making errors or missing something (the most common emotion/fear experienced by all new grads alike). Validate his feelings. Talk openly with him about this. Allow him to vent. Share your experience.

- Help him prioritize. Don't do it for him! Each morning, prioritize which patients he will see first and why. Help him anticipate what he will need before going into each patient's room.
- Discuss the focused assessment he will be performing for each patient. Ask him what system he will be focusing on and why. For example: If his patient is here for CHF, what will he be doing during his assessment? Review why a neuro and cranial nerve assessment are not necessary. Help him understand that by simply conversing with his patient, he *is* assessing neuro status. This actually might also be a good tip for Susie, TBH!
- Start giving him goals and timeframes to work through. Remember that short-term goal setting discussed previously? This is really beneficial for Sam. Review the table below and share this with him.

Patient Load	Assessment Time	Med Pass Time	Total Time Spent
1 patient	20 minutes	20 minutes	40 minutes
2 patients	15 minutes	20 minutes	70 minutes
3 patients	10 minutes	15 minutes	75 minutes
4 patients	10 minutes	15 minutes	100 minutes
5 patients	8 minutes	12 minutes	100 minutes

Cocky Cathy

Cathy. Cathy walks onto the unit like she's worked there 10 years. She doesn't ask many questions. Her time management is appropriate. You often hear her overdelegating to the techs on your unit. Oh, and receiving feedback isn't necessarily her cup of tea.

How to Deal

- Boundaries. Boundaries. Boundaries. It is crucial to set boundaries with Cathy at the beginning of orientation. It is vital that you explain to her that you will need to verify her competence in nursing skills before allowing her to fly solo in her patients' rooms. As Cathy's preceptor, you can watch her as many times as you need to until you are confident she is safe.
- Overconfidence is an indicator that Cathy is actually not as secure in nursing practice as she would like you to believe. Ask her questions about her plan of care. How is she going to prioritize? Why is she giving X medication? What does she anticipate happening next with her patient? These question allow you to assess and develop her nursing knowledge base.
- Be patient with Cathy and appreciate her confidence!
- Limit the praise you give Cathy before providing constructive feedback. She may not hear what you really need to say if you start with too much praise. She needs concise, direct feedback. Then move on.
- Do not be afraid to report ongoing problems to the facilitator of your orientation program.

It is likely Susie, Sam, and Cathy need a little extra TLC, and that is OK! We must remember that nursing is a beautiful profession comprised of unique personalities with different experiences and backgrounds. Every orientee you will precept will teach you a little more about yourself and help grow your coaching skills tenfold. Promise.

YOUR OWN EXPERIENCE

When I was a new graduate nurse, I made a mistake on my second day off of orientation. I acknowledged an order for a heparin drip and never got it started. With the way that the medication record was set up at the time, it was not a scheduled medication and fell out of sight after it was acknowledged. It was a busy day that got the best of me, and I woke up the next day to a voicemail from the charge nurse asking me why I never started the drip.

I was devastated. But I learned so much from this mistake. In fact, after a root cause analysis was conducted on this error, a major change was made in our electronic medication record that would prevent a heparin drip from ever being missed again.

To this day, this is a story I share openly with every nurse I precept. I saved this chapter for last because it might be the most important chapter you read. Sharing your own experiences, triumphs, and failures helps humanize nursing. It allows your orientees to understand that the feelings they are feeling are normal. It allows them to understand that they will make mistakes and that that will also grow from those mistakes. Share your story. Reflect with them. Not only will they learn from you and your experience, but you may find some healing and growth along the way.

STILL WITH ME, STUD?

I know you might be overwhelmed, as I have given you quite a few things to think about. But I want you to remember the way you used to admire your preceptor. The way he compassionately spoke with his patients. His effortless way of managing five patients seamlessly despite all the hiccups he faced. His calm demeanor in the middle of a storm.

So here's the thing.
You.Are.That.Person.Now.

You have evolved into a competent, more than capable nurse who is ready to inspire, mold, and grow each new nurse whose path you cross. Remember that your orientees are at the beginning of this path, where you once were, and need your help starting this journey.

- Support them always.
- Push them when you need to.
- Hold them accountable.
- Be kind.
- Be stern when you need to.
- Laugh with them.
- Grow with them.
- Be kind.
- Above all else, be their light.

As a preceptor, you've been offered to be a part of something pretty magical. The core development of a new nurse's journey is in the palm of your hands. What you do with this opportunity is up to you. But I promise, if you get your hands dirty, you won't regret it.

A toast to the preceptor tribe.
May we know them.
May we be them.
May we raise them.
You're gold, baby, solid gold.

Let's grow together,
Rachel.

ABOUT THE AUTHOR

Oh, hey there, Sunshine!

How are ya? My name is Rachel Edmondson, and I just wanted to pop in to say hello and introduce myself. I have worn quite a few hats in my (almost) five years of nursing to include bedside nurse, author, preceptor, charge nurse, nurse manager, bully-fighter, hand-holder, and blogger. I am a critical care nurse by trade, but I am now dabbling in a little bit of this and little of that on my hospital's Neuroscience and Orthopedic Floors.

I am a passionateer for reveling in the chaos and believe that together we are an unstoppable tribe. By chronicling my experiences in nursing, Nurse Tribe was born to connect and empower this beautiful community.

Thanks for connecting with me on this wild ride. It's my hope that you stay for awhile.

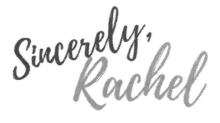

PS: For a wonderful book (written by Yours Truly) to give your new orientee check out *WWFD: A Real-World Guide to Surviving Nursing Orientation*. Available on Amazon or Nurseology.com.

32279571R00026

Made in the USA
Lexington, KY
01 March 2019